Understanding and Managing Lipedema

Empowering Women Through Knowledge, Treatment, and Support.

By Ernes Tech

Table of Content

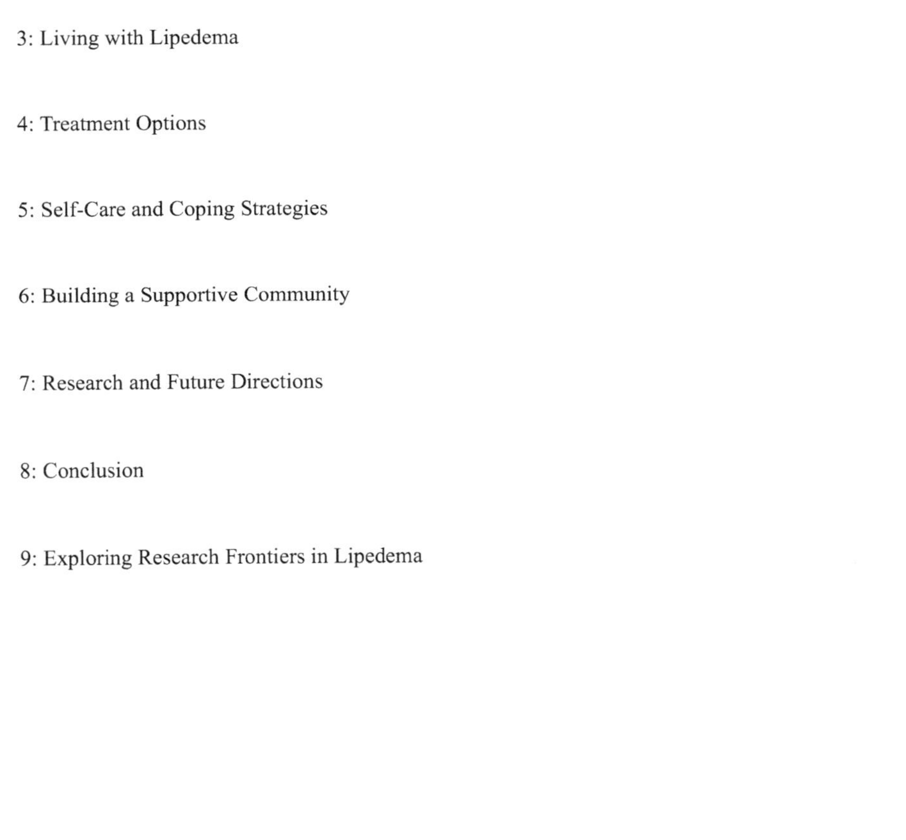

About the Author

E rnest is a dedicated advocate for health and wellness, focusing on empowering individuals living with chronic conditions. He brings expertise and firsthand experience to the topic of lipedema. Through our online platform, strive to raise awareness, provide support, and inspire others on their journey with lipedema.

Connect with Ernest to learn more about his work and join the community of individuals living well with lipedema.

About this Book

Please Note: This book is only intended for educational purposes, not for medical advice.

"Lipedema: Empowering Women Through Knowledge, Treatment, and Support" is a comprehensive guide that sheds light on the often misunderstood condition of lipedema. This book provides valuable insights into the challenges faced by women living with lipedema, a chronic disorder characterized by the abnormal accumulation of fat cells, typically in the legs and buttocks.

Written with empathy and expertise, this guide offers readers a deeper understanding of lipedema, its symptoms, and its impact on daily life. From diagnosis to treatment options, including conservative measures and surgical interventions, this book equips readers with the information they need to navigate their journey with confidence.

More than just a medical resource, "Lipedema: Empowering Women Through Knowledge, Treatment, and Support" emphasizes the importance of self-care, body positivity, and building a supportive community. Through inspiring stories, practical tips, and expert advice, readers will discover ways to manage their condition, advocate for their health needs, and embrace their unique beauty.

Whether you're a woman living with lipedema, a caregiver, or a healthcare professional, this book serves as a beacon of hope and empowerment. Join us on a journey of understanding, healing, and reclaiming control over your health and happiness.

1. Understanding Lipedema

Lipedema is a chronic condition characterized by the abnormal accumulation of fat cells, typically in the legs and buttocks, often causing pain, tenderness, and swelling. Despite being recognized for centuries, it remains widely misunderstood and underdiagnosed. In this chapter, we will delve into the fundamentals of lipedema, including its definition, signs and symptoms, and potential causes.

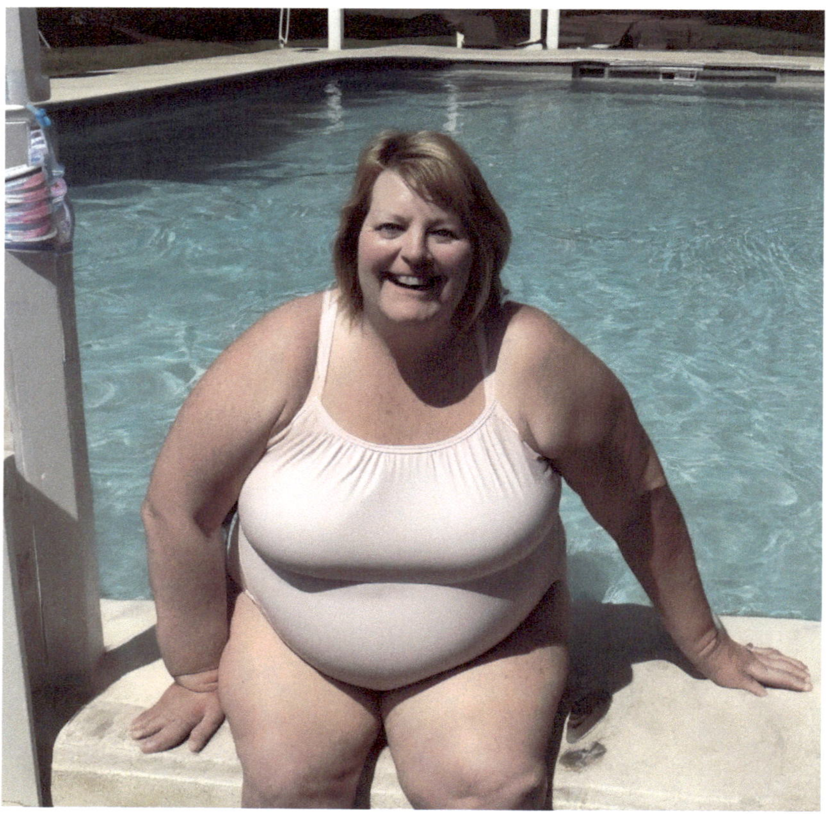

Defining Lipedema

Lipedema is a chronic disorder of adipose tissue distribution, primarily affecting women. It is characterized by symmetrically distributed excess fat, typically in the lower body, with sparing of the hands and feet. Unlike obesity, the fat accumulation in lipedema is disproportionate and resistant to diet and exercise. This condition often progresses over time, leading to pain, decreased mobility, and psychosocial distress.

Sources:
- Wold LE, Hines EA Jr, Allen EV. Lipedema of the legs; a syndrome characterized by fat legs and edema. Ann Intern Med. 1951;34(5):1243-50. [PubMed](https://pubmed.ncbi.nlm.nih.gov/14884326/)
- Herbst KL. Rare adipose disorders (RADs) masquerading as obesity. Acta Pharmacol Sin. 2012;33(2):155-72. [PubMed] (https://pubmed.ncbi.nlm.nih.gov/22301821/)

Signs and Symptoms

The hallmark signs of lipedema include:

1. Enlarged Lower Extremities: Excess fat deposition in the hips, thighs, and lower legs, often with a disproportionate appearance compared to the upper body.
2. Tenderness and Sensitivity: Affected areas may be tender to the touch and exhibit increased sensitivity to pressure.
3. Swelling (Edema): Edema, or fluid retention, is common in lipedema,

leading to swelling and discomfort, especially after prolonged standing or sitting.

4. Easy Bruising: Individuals with lipedema may bruise easily due to the fragility of blood vessels in affected areas.

5. Pain and Discomfort: Many people with lipedema experience pain, ranging from mild discomfort to severe, debilitating pain, often exacerbated by physical activity or pressure on the affected areas.

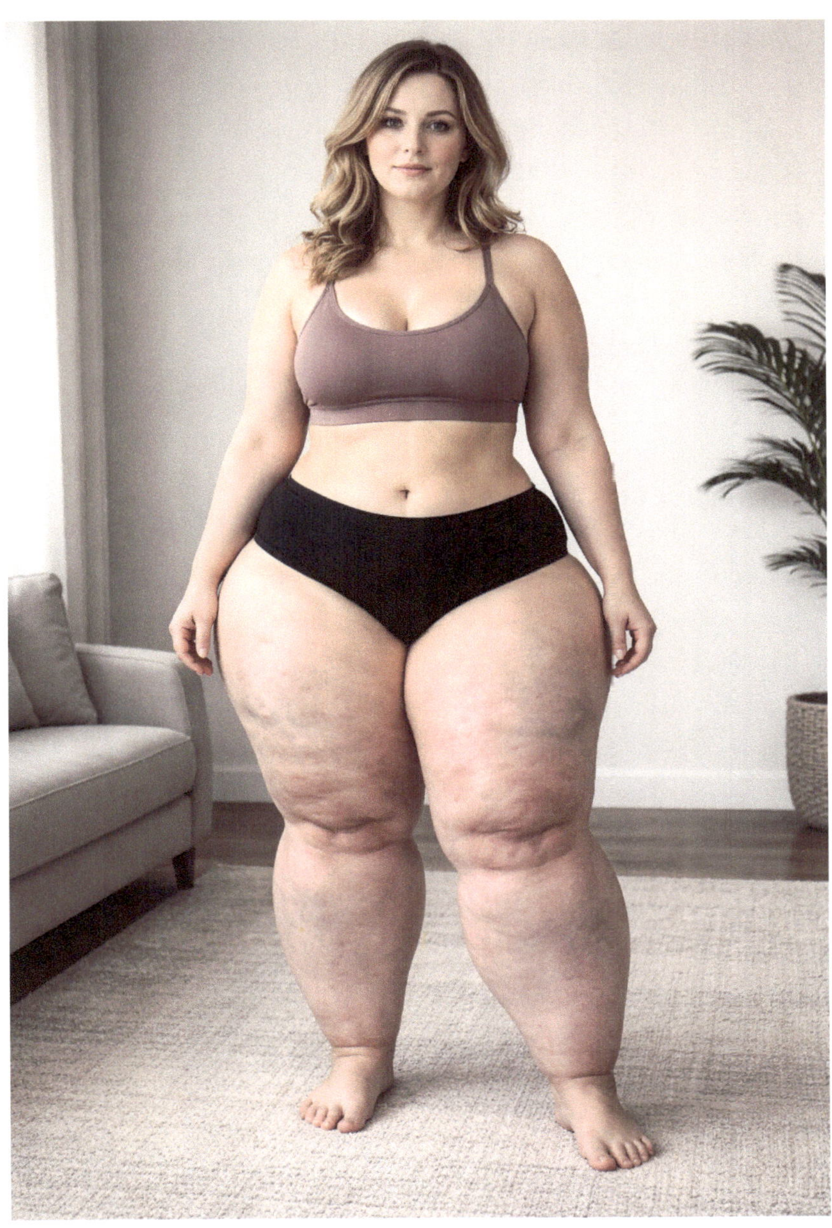

Sources:

- Forner-Cordero I, Szolnoky G, Forner-Cordero A, Kemény L. Lipedema: an

overview of its clinical manifestations, diagnosis and treatment of the disproportional fatty deposition syndrome - systematic review. Clin Obes. 2012;2(3-4):86-95. [PubMed](https://pubmed.ncbi.nlm.nih.gov/25586579/)
- Al-Ghadban S, Cromer W, Allen M, Ussery C, Badowski M, Harris D, et al. Dilated blood and lymphatic microvessels, angiogenesis, increased macrophages, and adipocyte hypertrophy in lipedema thigh skin and fat tissue. J Obes. 2019;2019:8747461. [PubMed]
(https://pubmed.ncbi.nlm.nih.gov/31467815/)

Causes and Risk Factors

The exact cause of lipedema remains unclear, but several factors may contribute to its development, including genetics, hormonal influences, and metabolic dysfunction. Lipedema primarily affects women, suggesting a hormonal component, with onset typically occurring around puberty, pregnancy, or menopause. Genetic predisposition may also play a role, as lipedema often runs in families. Additionally, hormonal fluctuations, such as those associated with estrogen and progesterone, may exacerbate symptoms and contribute to disease progression.

Sources:
- Child AH, Gordon KD, Sharpe P, Brice G, Ostergaard P, Jeffery S, et al. Lipedema: an inherited condition. Am J Med Genet A. 2010;152A(4):970-6. [PubMed](https://pubmed.ncbi.nlm.nih.gov/20358590/)
- Szél E, Kemény L, Groma G, Szolnoky G. Pathophysiological dilemmas of lipedema. Med Hypotheses. 2014;83(5):599-606. [PubMed]
(https://pubmed.ncbi.nlm.nih.gov/25257071/)

Understanding the basics of lipedema is crucial for early recognition, accurate diagnosis, and effective management of this condition. Stay tuned for the next chapter, where we'll explore the diagnostic process and how to recognize the signs of lipedema.

2. Diagnosing Lipedema

Diagnosing lipedema can be challenging due to its similarity to other conditions such as obesity, lymphedema, and venous insufficiency. However, early recognition and accurate diagnosis are essential for initiating appropriate treatment and improving patients' quality of life. In this chapter, we will explore the diagnostic process for lipedema, including recognizing the signs, undergoing a medical evaluation, and considering differential diagnoses.

Recognizing the Signs

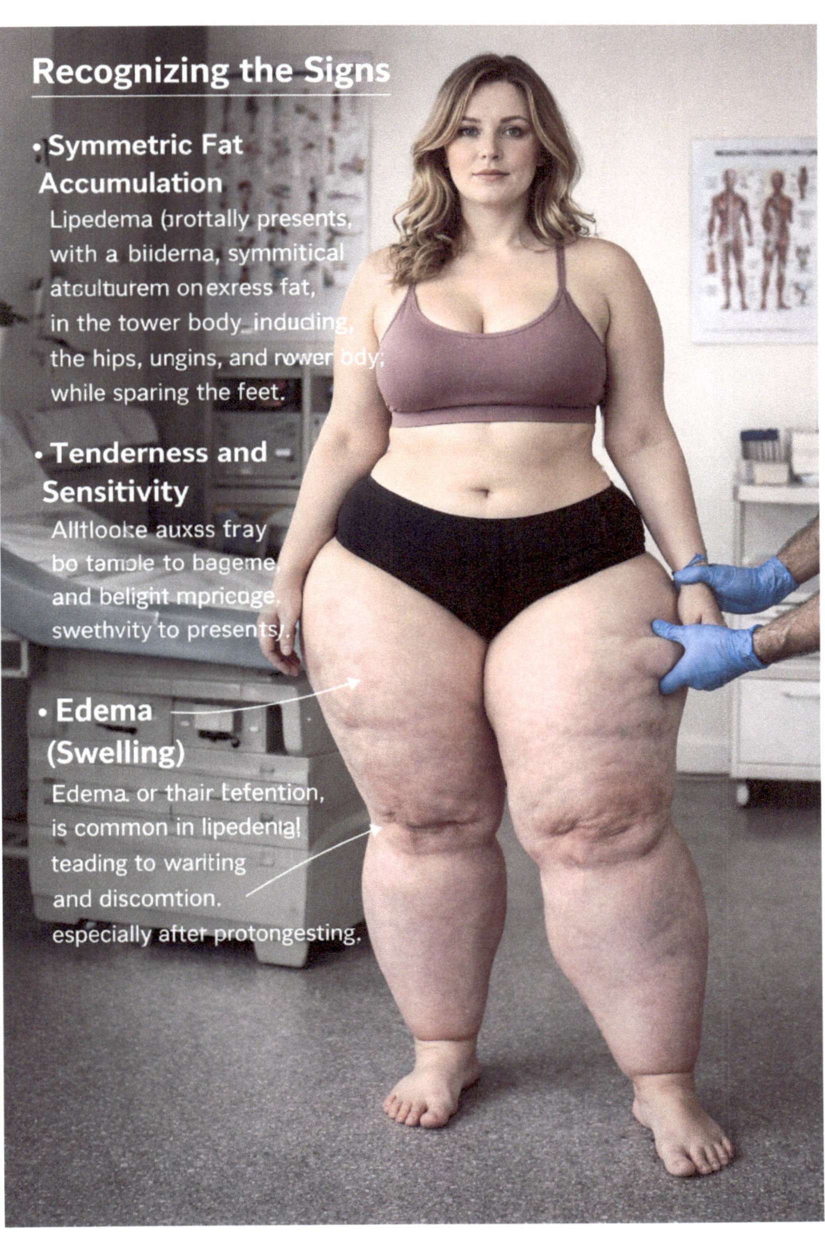

- **Symmetric Fat Accumulation**
  Lipedema typically presents, with a bilateral, symmetrical accumulation of excess fat, in the lower body, including, the hips, thighs, and lower body; while sparing the feet.

- **Tenderness and Sensitivity**
  Affected areas may be tender to the touch, and may experience increased sensitivity to pressure.

- **Edema (Swelling)**
  Edema, or fluid retention, is common in lipedema, leading to swelling and discomfort, especially after prolonged sitting.

Recognizing the Signs

The diagnosis of lipedema begins with recognizing the characteristic signs and symptoms associated with the condition. Clinicians should be vigilant for the following features:

1. Symmetric Fat Accumulation: Lipedema typically presents with a bilateral, symmetrical distribution of excess fat in the lower body, including the hips, thighs, and lower legs, while sparing the feet.

2. Tenderness and Sensitivity: Affected areas may be tender to the touch and exhibit increased sensitivity to pressure, distinguishing lipedema from simple obesity.

3. Edema (Swelling): Edema, or fluid retention, is common in lipedema, leading to swelling and discomfort, especially after prolonged standing or sitting.

4. Easy Bruising: Individuals with lipedema may bruise easily due to the fragility of blood vessels in affected areas, known as easy bruising or ecchymosis.

5. Pain and Discomfort: Many people with lipedema experience pain, ranging from mild discomfort to severe, debilitating pain, often exacerbated by physical activity or pressure on the affected areas.

Sources:
- Wold LE, Hines EA Jr, Allen EV. Lipedema of the legs; a syndrome characterized by fat legs and edema. Ann Intern Med. 1951;34(5):1243-50. [PubMed](https://pubmed.ncbi.nlm.nih.gov/14884326/)
- Forner-Cordero I, Szolnoky G, Forner-Cordero A, Kemény L. Lipedema: an

overview of its clinical manifestations, diagnosis and treatment of the disproportional fatty deposition syndrome - systematic review. Clin Obes. 2012;2(3-4):86-95. [PubMed](https://pubmed.ncbi.nlm.nih.gov/25586579/)

Medical Evaluation and Diagnosis

A comprehensive medical evaluation is essential for confirming the diagnosis of lipedema and ruling out other conditions. This evaluation may include:

1. Medical History: The clinician will inquire about the patient's medical history, including symptoms, onset, progression, and family history of lipedema or related conditions.

2. Physical Examination: A thorough physical examination will be performed to assess the distribution of fat, tenderness, swelling, and other signs suggestive of lipedema.

3. Diagnostic Tests: While there are no specific diagnostic tests for lipedema, imaging studies such as ultrasound or MRI may be used to evaluate fat distribution and rule out other conditions such as lymphedema or venous insufficiency.

Differential Diagnosis

Several conditions may mimic the signs and symptoms of lipedema, making it important to consider differential diagnoses. These may include:

1. Obesity: Simple obesity may present with similar features of fat accumulation, but typically lacks the characteristic tenderness and sensitivity seen in lipedema.

2. Lymphedema: Lymphedema involves swelling due to impaired lymphatic drainage, often affecting one limb more than the other and accompanied by pitting edema.

3. Venous Insufficiency: Venous insufficiency may cause leg swelling and discomfort, but typically presents with varicose veins and skin changes such as stasis dermatitis.

Accurate diagnosis is the cornerstone of effective management for individuals with lipedema. By recognizing the signs, conducting a thorough medical evaluation, and considering differential diagnoses, healthcare professionals can provide timely and appropriate care for patients with this condition. Stay tuned for the next chapter, where we'll explore treatment options for lipedema.

3. Living with Lipedema

Living with lipedema can present significant challenges, both physically and emotionally. In this chapter, we will explore the impact of lipedema on daily life, including the physical symptoms, emotional toll, and strategies for coping with this chronic condition.

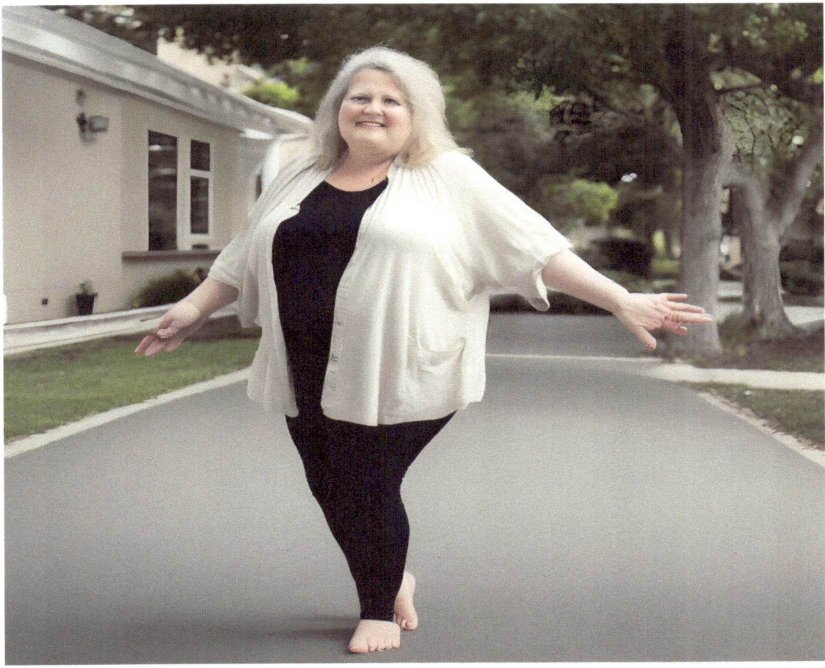

Impact on Daily Life

Lipedema can have a profound impact on various aspects of daily life, including:

1. Mobility: The excess weight and swelling associated with lipedema can impair mobility, making it difficult to perform daily activities such as walking, standing, or climbing stairs.

2. Pain and Discomfort: Many individuals with lipedema experience pain and discomfort, ranging from mild aches to severe, debilitating pain, which can interfere with work, exercise, and sleep.

3. Body Image and Self-Esteem: Lipedema can negatively impact body image and self-esteem due to the visible changes in body shape and the perception of being "different" from others.

4. Clothing Challenges: Finding clothing that fits comfortably and accommodates the disproportionate fat distribution characteristic of lipedema can be challenging and frustrating.

5. Social and Emotional Well-Being: Coping with the physical and emotional challenges of lipedema can lead to social isolation, depression, anxiety, and other mental health issues.

Sources:

- Herbst KL. Rare adipose disorders (RADs) masquerading as obesity. Acta Pharmacol Sin. 2012;33(2):155-72. [PubMed] (https://pubmed.ncbi.nlm.nih.gov/22301821/)
- Buck DW 2nd, Herbst KL. Lipedema: a relatively common disease with extremely common misconceptions. Plast Reconstr Surg Glob Open. 2016;4(9):e1043. [PubMed](https://pubmed.ncbi.nlm.nih.gov/27757353/)

Emotional and Psychological Effects

The emotional toll of living with lipedema can be significant, leading to feelings of frustration, embarrassment, shame, and despair. Common emotional and psychological effects of lipedema include:

1. Depression and Anxiety: Coping with the physical limitations, pain, and changes in body image associated with lipedema can contribute to depression and anxiety.

2. Social Isolation: Many individuals with lipedema may withdraw from social activities and relationships due to feelings of self-consciousness and fear of judgment.

3. Negative Body Image: Lipedema can distort body image and lead to dissatisfaction with one's appearance, impacting self-esteem and confidence.

4. Stress and Coping Mechanisms: Managing the challenges of living with lipedema can be stressful, leading some individuals to engage in unhealthy coping mechanisms such as emotional eating or avoidance behaviors.

Sources:
- Reich-Schupke S, Schmeller W, Brauer WJ, Hinrichs R, Stücker M. Psychological factors in patients with lipedema - a nationwide survey in Germany. J Dtsch Dermatol Ges. 2017;15(12):1180-1185. [PubMed] (https://pubmed.ncbi.nlm.nih.gov/28940405/)
- Cheville AL, Tchou J. Barriers to rehabilitation following surgery for primary or secondary lymphedema: A review of the literature. Rehabil Oncol. 2008;26(1):29-35. [PubMed](https://pubmed.ncbi.nlm.nih.gov/18025588/)

Coping Strategies

Despite the challenges of living with lipedema, there are strategies that individuals can employ to improve their quality of life and well-being:

1. Seeking Support: Connecting with others who understand the challenges of living with lipedema through support groups, online communities, or counseling can provide valuable emotional support and encouragement.

2. Practicing Self-Care: Engaging in self-care activities such as gentle exercise, massage, compression therapy, and mindfulness techniques can help manage pain, reduce stress, and improve overall well-being.

3. Advocating for Yourself: Advocating for proper diagnosis, treatment, and support from healthcare providers is essential for effectively managing lipedema and improving quality of life.

4. Educating Others: Raising awareness and educating others about lipedema can help combat stigma and promote understanding and acceptance within the community.

Living with lipedema presents unique challenges, but with support, self-care, and advocacy, individuals can learn to manage their symptoms and improve their quality of life. Stay tuned for the next chapter, where we'll explore treatment options for lipedema.

4. Treatment Options

Effective management of lipedema involves a multifaceted approach aimed at reducing symptoms, improving quality of life, and preventing disease progression. In this chapter, we will explore the various treatment options available for individuals living with lipedema, including conservative measures, medical interventions, and surgical procedures.

Conservative Management

1. Lifestyle Modifications: Adopting healthy lifestyle habits such as maintaining a balanced diet, staying hydrated, and engaging in regular physical activity can help manage weight and reduce symptoms of lipedema.

Conservative Management

1. Lifestyle Modifications:

Adopting healthy lifestyle habits such as maintaining a balanced diet, staying hydrated, and engaging in regular physical activity can help manage weight and reduce symptoms of lipedema.

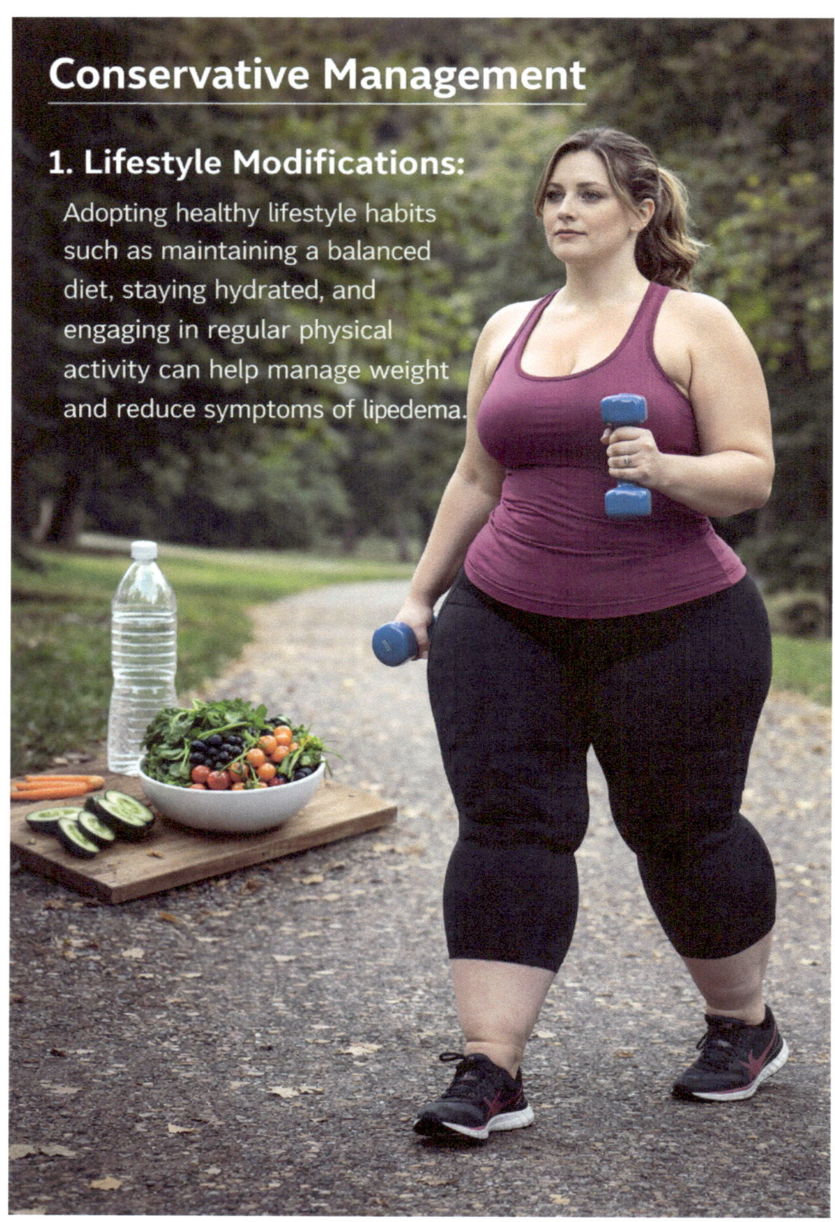

2. Compression Therapy: Wearing compression garments, such as compression stockings or wraps, can help reduce swelling, improve lymphatic flow, and alleviate discomfort associated with lipedema.

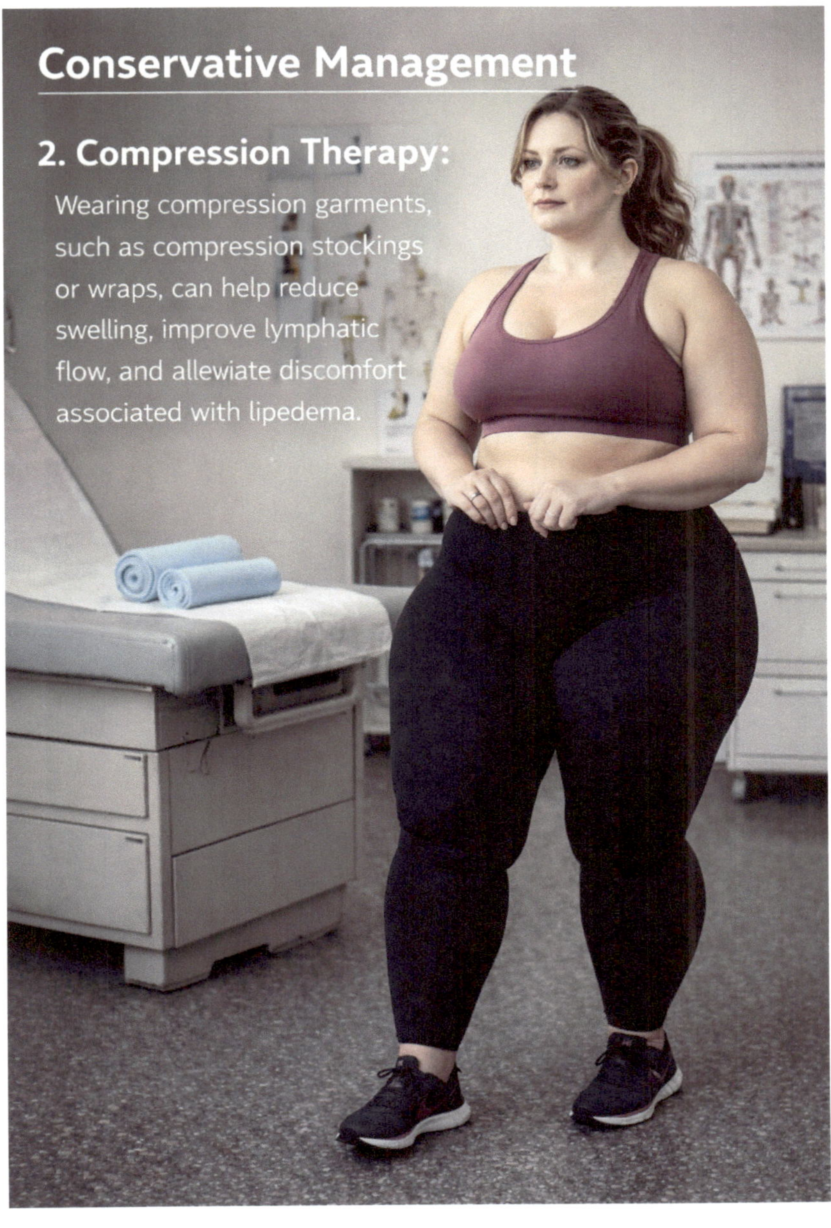

3. Manual Lymphatic Drainage (MLD): MLD is a specialized massage technique performed by trained therapists to stimulate lymphatic drainage, reduce swelling, and improve circulation in affected areas.

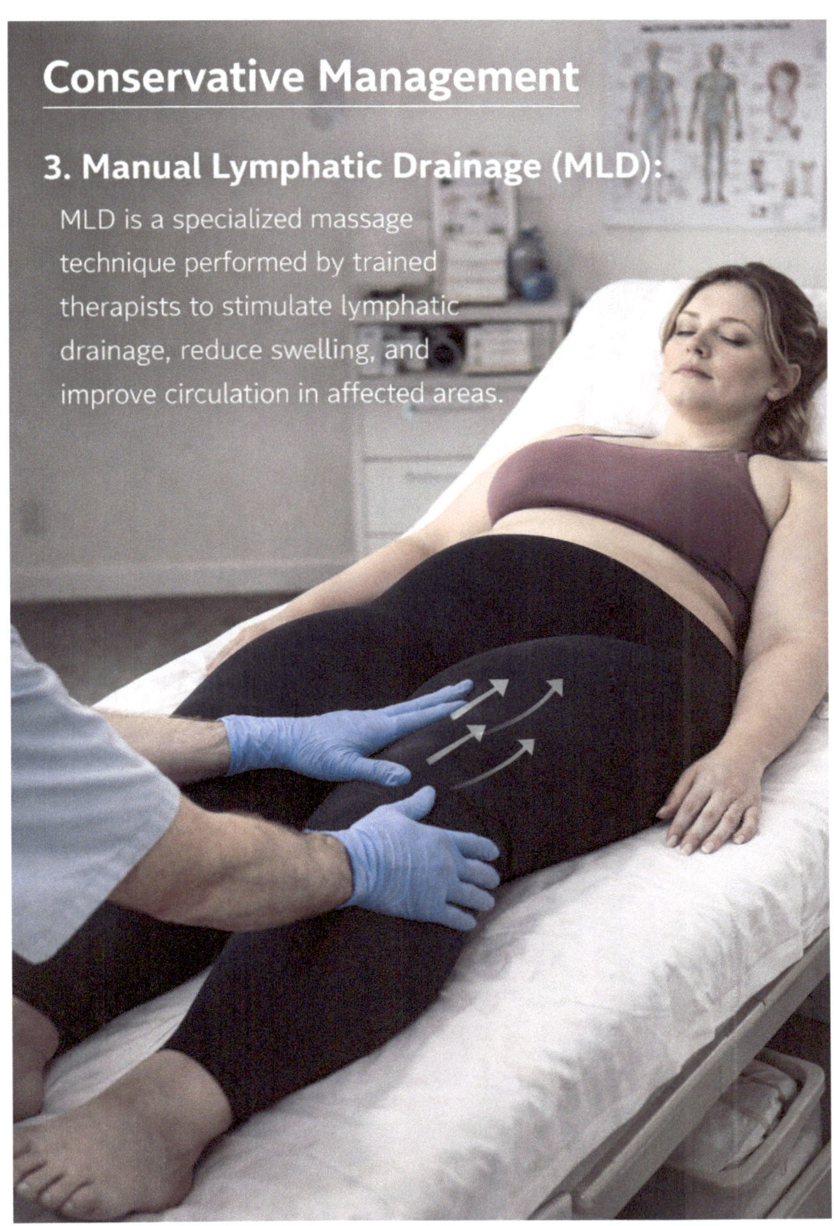

4. Exercise and Physical Therapy: Participating in low-impact exercises such as swimming, walking, or cycling, as well as targeted physical therapy exercises, can help improve mobility, muscle tone, and overall well-being.

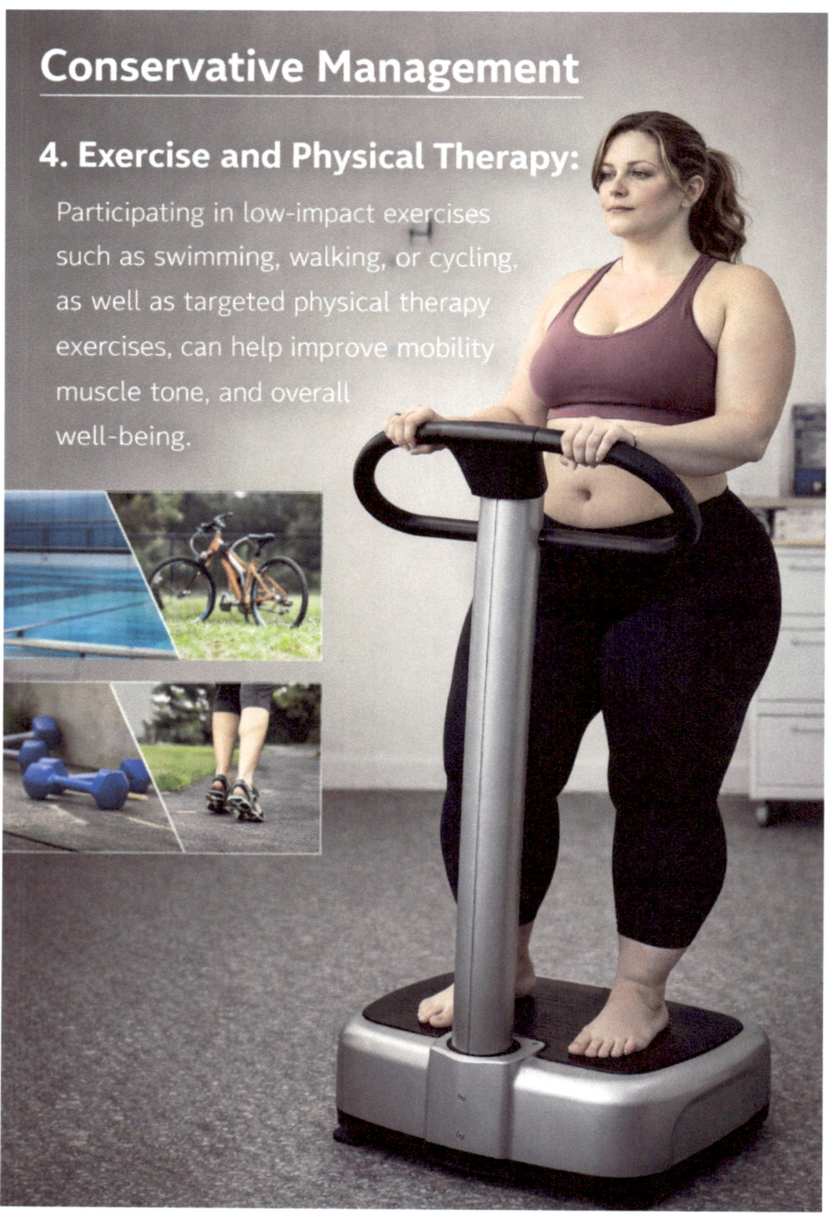

Sources:

- Forner-Cordero I, Szolnoky G, Forner-Cordero A, Kemény L. Lipedema: an overview of its clinical manifestations, diagnosis and treatment of the disproportional fatty deposition syndrome - systematic review. Clin Obes. 2012;2(3-4):86-95. [PubMed](https://pubmed.ncbi.nlm.nih.gov/25586579/)
- Szél E, Kemény L, Groma G, Szolnoky G. Pathophysiological dilemmas of lipedema. Med Hypotheses. 2014;83(5):599-606. [PubMed] (https://pubmed.ncbi.nlm.nih.gov/25257071/)

Medical Interventions (Only when necessary)

1. Medications: Certain medications, such as diuretics, lymphatic stimulants, and anti-inflammatory drugs, may be prescribed to help reduce swelling, alleviate pain, and improve lymphatic function in individuals with lipedema. But for you go this route, you should make sure that you are healed from within, control your diet and mindfullness, seek help from the Docker if needed.

2. Tumescent Liposuction: Tumescent liposuction is a surgical procedure performed under local anesthesia to remove excess fat deposits characteristic of lipedema, reducing pain, swelling, and improving mobility and body contour.

3. Debulking Surgery: Debulking surgery involves the removal of large, fibrotic masses of adipose tissue in severely affected areas, typically performed in combination with liposuction to achieve optimal results.

4. Lymphatic Surgery: Lymphatic surgery, such as lymphovenous anastomosis or lymph node transfer, may be considered for individuals with advanced lipedema and associated lymphatic dysfunction to improve lymphatic drainage and reduce swelling.

Sources:

- Stutz JJ, Krahl D. Water-assisted liposuction for patients with lipoedema: histologic and immunohistologic analysis of the aspirates of 30 lipoedema patients. Aesthetic Plast Surg. 2009;33(2):153-62. [PubMed] (https://pubmed.ncbi.nlm.nih.gov/19172238/)
- Herbst KL. Rare adipose disorders (RADs) masquerading as obesity. Acta Pharmacol Sin. 2012;33(2):155-72. [PubMed] (https://pubmed.ncbi.nlm.nih.gov/22301821/)

Treatment options for lipedema should be individualized based on the severity of symptoms, patient preferences, and available resources. By combining conservative measures, medical interventions, and surgical procedures, individuals with lipedema can effectively manage their condition and improve their quality of life. Stay tuned for the next chapter, where we'll explore self-care strategies and coping mechanisms for living with lipedema.

5. Self-Care and Coping Strategies

L iving with lipedema can be challenging, but there are strategies individuals can employ to improve their quality of life and well-being. In this chapter, we will explore self-care practices and coping strategies that can help individuals manage the physical and emotional impact of lipedema.

Embracing Body Positivity

1. Acceptance and Self-Love: Embracing body positivity involves accepting and loving oneself, regardless of physical appearance or perceived flaws. Practicing self-compassion and gratitude can help individuals cultivate a positive body image and improve self-esteem.

Sources:
- Neff KD, Vonk R. Self-compassion versus global self-esteem: two different ways of relating to oneself. J Pers. 2009;77(1):23-50. [PubMed] (https://pubmed.ncbi.nlm.nih.gov/19076989/)

Practicing Self-Care

1. Mindfulness and Relaxation Techniques: Engaging in mindfulness meditation, deep breathing exercises, or progressive muscle relaxation can help reduce stress, promote relaxation, and improve overall well-being.

2. Gentle Exercise: Participating in low-impact exercises such as yoga, swimming, or tai chi can help improve mobility, reduce pain, and enhance mood without exacerbating symptoms of lipedema.

Follow the steps below for gentle excecises:

1. Preparation: Find a quiet and comfortable space to practice yoga. Wear loose, breathable clothing that allows for easy movement.

   Place a yoga mat or a non-slip surface on the floor to provide cushioning and stability.

2. Warm-Up: Begin with a gentle warm-up to prepare your body for exercise and increase blood flow to the muscles.

   You can start by standing tall with feet hip-width apart and gently roll your shoulders backward and forward.

   Then, perform gentle neck stretches, side stretches, and arm circles to loosen up.

3. Basic Poses: Choose a few basic yoga poses that focus on stretching and strengthening the body while being mindful of your limitations and
   comfort level. Some suitable poses for individuals with lipedema include:

   - Mountain Pose (Tadasana): Stand tall with feet together or hip-width apart, arms by your sides, and palms facing forward. Engage your core, lengthen your
     spine, and relax your shoulders. This pose helps improve posture and alignment.

   - Child's Pose (Balasana): Kneel on the mat with toes touching and knees hip-width apart. Lower your hips back toward your heels and extend your arms forward,
     resting your forehead on the mat. This pose gently stretches the back, hips,

and thighs, promoting relaxation.

   - Seated Forward Fold (Paschimottanasana): Sit on the mat with legs extended in front of you. Inhale to lengthen your spine, then exhale as you hinge forward from
   the hips, reaching toward your toes or shins. Keep your back straight and avoid rounding your spine. This pose stretches the hamstrings and lower back.

   - Supported Bridge Pose: Lie on your back with knees bent and feet hip-width apart. Place a yoga block or rolled-up towel under your sacrum
   (the triangular bone at the base of your spine). Relax your arms by your sides and breathe deeply. This pose helps relieve tension in the lower back and hips.

4. Breathing: Focus on your breath throughout the practice, inhaling deeply through the nose and exhaling slowly through the mouth.
   Use your breath to cultivate a sense of calm and relaxation, allowing it to guide you through each movement.

5. Mindfulness: Practice mindfulness by paying attention to sensations in your body, thoughts, and emotions as you move through each pose.
   Notice any areas of tension or discomfort and adjust accordingly, never pushing yourself into pain.

6. Cool Down and Relaxation: Finish your gentle yoga session with a few minutes of relaxation in Savasana (Corpse Pose).
   Lie on your back with arms and legs extended, palms facing up, and eyes closed. Allow your body to fully relax,
   releasing any remaining tension.

7. Hydration and Rest: Drink water to stay hydrated after your practice, and take time to rest and rejuvenate. Listen to your body and

    honor its needs for recovery.

By following these steps and practicing gentle yoga regularly, individuals with lipedema can experience improved mobility, reduced pain, and enhanced well-being without exacerbating symptoms. It's important to approach exercise with patience, compassion, and awareness of your body's limitations.

Sources:

- Zgierska A, Rabago D, Chawla N, Kushner K, Koehler R, Marlatt A. Mindfulness meditation for substance use disorders: a systematic review. Subst Abus. 2009;30(4):266-94. [PubMed] (https://pubmed.ncbi.nlm.nih.gov/19904664/)

Building a Supportive Community

1. Seeking Support: Connecting with others who understand the challenges of living with lipedema through support groups, online communities,

    or counseling can provide valuable emotional support and encouragement.

[Tip]: For Support Contact us via Email to connect you with the community: lipedema@ernestech.com

Here is how to go about seeking support:

Research Support Options: Start by researching different support options available for individuals living with lipedema. This can include support groups, online communities, counseling services, or forums dedicated to discussing the condition. Look for reputable organizations, websites, or healthcare providers specializing in lipedema for reliable information and resources.

Identify Suitable Support Groups: Search for local support groups or online communities specifically tailored to individuals with lipedema. These groups provide a safe space for sharing experiences, asking questions, and receiving support from others who understand the challenges of living with the condition. Websites like Meetup, Facebook groups, or forums dedicated to lipedema can be valuable resources for finding relevant support groups.

Join Support Groups: Once you've identified suitable support groups, take the step to join them. This may involve signing up for in-person support group meetings or requesting to join online communities or forums. Many online support groups have membership approval processes to ensure the safety and privacy of members.

Introduce Yourself: After joining a support group or online community, introduce yourself to other members. Share a brief overview of your experience with lipedema, including any challenges you're facing or goals you're working towards. This helps establish connections with fellow members and opens the door for further discussions and support.

Participate Actively: Engage actively in support group activities and discussions. Offer support and encouragement to others sharing their experiences, and don't hesitate to ask questions or seek advice when needed. Sharing your own insights and coping strategies can also be helpful to fellow members facing similar challenges.

Attend Meetings or Events: If you've joined an in-person support group, make an effort to attend meetings or events regularly. These gatherings provide opportunities for face-to-face interactions, building deeper connections with fellow members, and gaining additional support and insights.

Seek Professional Support: In addition to peer support groups, consider seeking professional support through counseling or therapy. A mental health professional experienced in working with individuals living with chronic conditions like lipedema can provide valuable emotional support, coping strategies, and guidance for managing the psychological aspects of the condition.

Practice Self-Care: While seeking support from others is important, don't forget to prioritize self-care. Take time for activities that bring you joy and relaxation, practice mindfulness and stress-reduction techniques, and prioritize your physical and emotional well-being.

By following these steps and actively seeking support from peer groups, online communities, counseling services, and other resources, individuals living with lipedema can find valuable emotional support, encouragement, and understanding from others who share similar experiences. Remember that seeking support is a sign of strength, and you're not alone in your journey with lipedema.

Seeking Support

Researching and Joining Support Groups

Individuals living with lipedema can find valuable emotional support through peer groups, online communities. and **counseling** services.

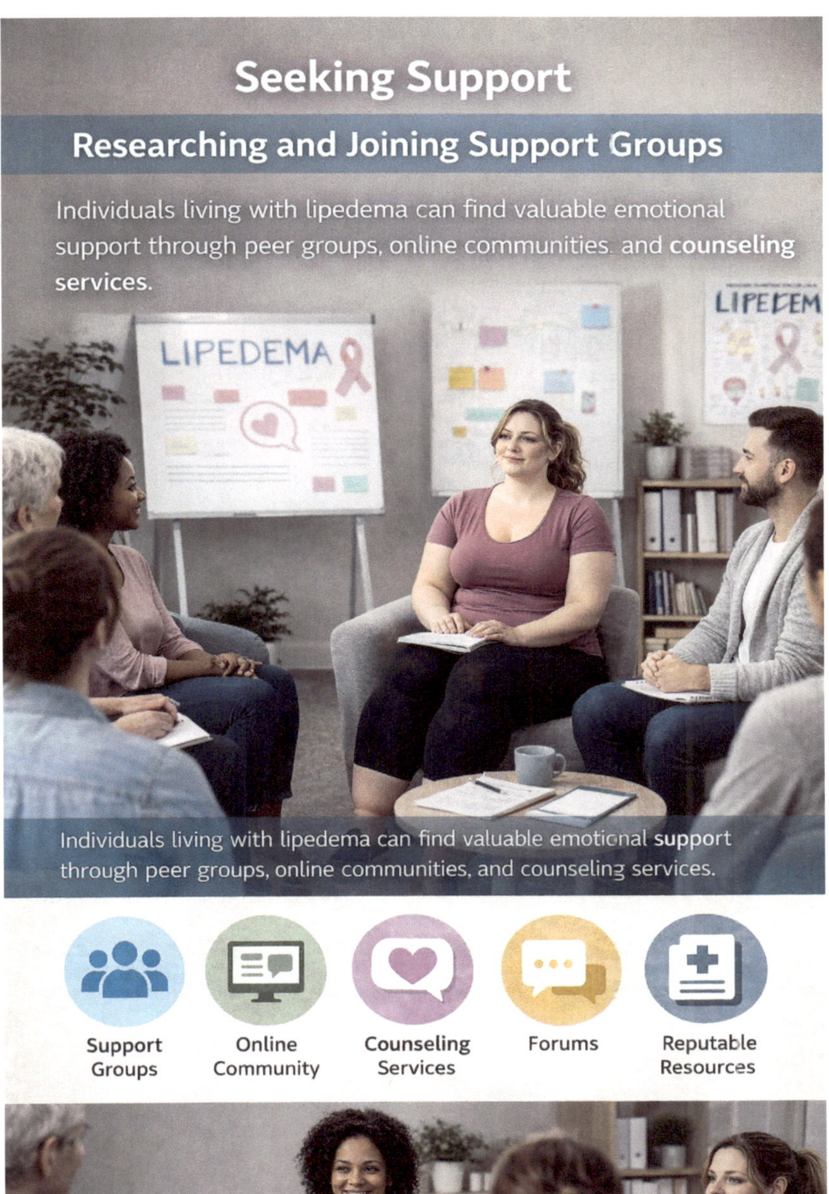

2. Sharing Experiences: Sharing experiences, insights, and coping strategies with others who have lipedema can help reduce feelings of isolation and promote a sense of belonging and validation.

Sources:

- Reich-Schupke S, Schmeller W, Brauer WJ, Hinrichs R, Stücker M. Psychological factors in patients with lipedema - a nationwide survey in Germany. J Dtsch Dermatol Ges. 2017;15(12):1180-1185. [PubMed] (https://pubmed.ncbi.nlm.nih.gov/28940405/)

Advocating for Yourself

1. Educating Others: Raising awareness and educating others about lipedema can help combat stigma and promote understanding and acceptance within the community.

2. Seeking Treatment: Advocating for proper diagnosis, treatment, and support from healthcare providers is essential for effectively managing lipedema and improving quality of life.

Sources:

- Cheville AL, Tchou J. Barriers to rehabilitation following surgery for primary or secondary lymphedema: A review of the literature. Rehabil Oncol. 2008;26(1):29-35. [PubMed](https://pubmed.ncbi.nlm.nih.gov/18025588/)

By practicing self-care, seeking support, and advocating for themselves, individuals with lipedema can enhance their well-being and cope more effectively with the challenges of living with this condition. Stay tuned for the next chapter, where we'll explore ongoing research and future directions in the treatment of lipedema.

6. Building a Supportive Community

L iving with lipedema can feel isolating, but finding a supportive community can provide comfort, understanding, and encouragement. In this chapter, we'll explore the importance of building a supportive community and how individuals with lipedema can connect with others for emotional support, practical advice, and empowerment.

Connecting with Others

1. Support Groups: Joining local or online support groups specifically for individuals with lipedema can provide a safe space to share experiences, ask questions, and offer support to one another.

2. Online Communities: Engaging with online communities, forums, and social media groups dedicated to lipedema can help individuals connect with others who understand their experiences and provide valuable insights and resources.

Sources:
- Lipedema Foundation - [Support Groups]https://lipedema.org/support-groups/)
- Lipedema Project - [Online Community] (https://www.lipedemaproject.org/community/)

Sharing Experiences

1. Storytelling: Sharing personal stories, challenges, and triumphs with lipedema can help individuals feel heard, validated, and understood by others who may be going through similar experiences.

2. Peer Support: Offering support and encouragement to fellow community members can foster a sense of belonging, empowerment, and resilience among individuals with lipedema.

Sources:
- Lipedema Project - [Share Your Story]
(https://www.lipedemaproject.org/share-your-story/)

Advocacy and Awareness

1. Raising Awareness: Participating in advocacy efforts, awareness campaigns, and fundraising events for lipedema can help educate the public, healthcare professionals, and policymakers about the challenges faced by individuals with this condition.

2. Empowering Others: Empowering fellow community members to advocate for themselves, seek proper diagnosis and treatment, and access resources and support can create a ripple effect of positive change within the lipedema community.

Sources:
- International Lymphedema & Lipedema Society (ILF) - [Advocacy]
(https://www.lipedema.org/advocacy/)

Seeking Professional Guidance

1. Expert Advice: Consulting with healthcare professionals, patient advocates, or lipedema specialists can provide individuals with accurate information, personalized guidance, and access to appropriate resources and treatment options.

2. Collaborative Care: Building a collaborative relationship with healthcare providers who are knowledgeable about lipedema can empower individuals to advocate for their needs, make informed decisions, and achieve better health outcomes.

Sources:
- Lipedema Foundation - [Find a Doctor](https://lipedema.org/find-a-doctor/)

By building a supportive community, individuals with lipedema can find strength, solidarity, and empowerment in their journey of living with this condition. Stay tuned for the next chapter, where we'll explore ongoing research and future directions in the treatment of lipedema.

7. Research and Future Directions

Research into lipedema is ongoing, with scientists and healthcare professionals striving to better understand the underlying causes, improve diagnostic methods, and develop more effective treatments for this condition. In this chapter, we'll explore the current state of research on lipedema and potential future directions in the field.

Current Research Landscape

1. Genetic Studies: Researchers are investigating the genetic factors that may contribute to the development of lipedema, aiming to identify specific gene mutations or variants associated with the condition.

2. Pathophysiological Mechanisms: Studies are exploring the underlying pathophysiological mechanisms of lipedema, including inflammation, adipose tissue dysfunction, lymphatic abnormalities, and hormonal influences.

Sources:
- Child AH, Gordon KD, Sharpe P, Brice G, Ostergaard P, Jeffery S, et al. Lipedema: an inherited condition. Am J Med Genet A. 2010;152A(4):970-6. [PubMed](https://pubmed.ncbi.nlm.nih.gov/20358590/)
- Szél E, Kemény L, Groma G, Szolnoky G. Pathophysiological dilemmas of lipedema. Med Hypotheses. 2014;83(5):599-606. [PubMed] (https://pubmed.ncbi.nlm.nih.gov/25257071/)

Clinical Studies

1. Treatment Trials: Clinical trials are evaluating the safety and efficacy of various treatment modalities for lipedema, including medications, compression therapy, surgical interventions, and novel therapeutic approaches.

2. Patient Outcomes: Researchers are conducting longitudinal studies to assess patient-reported outcomes, quality of life, functional status, and satisfaction with different treatment options for lipedema.

Sources:
- Forner-Cordero I, Szolnoky G, Forner-Cordero A, Kemény L. Lipedema: an overview of its clinical manifestations, diagnosis and treatment of the disproportional fatty deposition syndrome - systematic review. Clin Obes. 2012;2(3-4):86-95. [PubMed](https://pubmed.ncbi.nlm.nih.gov/25586579/)
- Buck DW 2nd, Herbst KL. Lipedema: a relatively common disease with extremely common misconceptions. Plast Reconstr Surg Glob Open. 2016;4(9):e1043. [PubMed](https://pubmed.ncbi.nlm.nih.gov/27757353/)

Future Directions

1. Precision Medicine: Advancements in genomic medicine may lead to personalized treatment approaches for lipedema, tailored to an individual's genetic profile, underlying pathophysiology, and specific clinical needs.

2. Targeted Therapies: Research into novel therapeutic targets and treatment modalities, such as pharmacological agents targeting adipose tissue dysfunction or inflammation, may offer new avenues for the management of lipedema.

Sources:

- Herbst KL. Rare adipose disorders (RADs) masquerading as obesity. Acta Pharmacol Sin. 2012;33(2):155-72. [PubMed] (https://pubmed.ncbi.nlm.nih.gov/22301821/

- Zuercher JN, Cummins KA, Anstey KL. Targeting inflammation in lipedema: a review of current treatments. Cutis. 2021;107(2):E10-E15. [PubMed] (https://pubmed.ncbi.nlm.nih.gov/34486974/)

Participating in Research

1. Clinical Trials: Individuals with lipedema may have the opportunity to participate in clinical trials investigating new treatments, diagnostic tools, or research studies aimed at advancing our understanding of the condition.

2. Patient Advocacy: Advocating for increased research funding, collaboration among researchers, and inclusion of lipedema in research agendas can help drive progress in the field and improve outcomes for individuals with the condition.

Sources:

- Lipedema Foundation - [Research](https://lipedema.org/research/)

As research into lipedema continues to evolve, there is hope for improved diagnostic methods, more effective treatments, and better outcomes for individuals living with this condition. By staying informed, advocating for research funding, and participating in clinical trials, individuals with lipedema can play an active role in shaping the future of care for themselves and others affected by this condition.

8. Conclusion

I n this comprehensive guide to living with lipedema, we have explored the multifaceted aspects of this chronic condition, from its definition and diagnosis to treatment options, self-care strategies, and ongoing research. Lipedema presents unique challenges, both physical and emotional, but with knowledge, support, and proactive management, individuals can navigate their journey with resilience and empowerment.

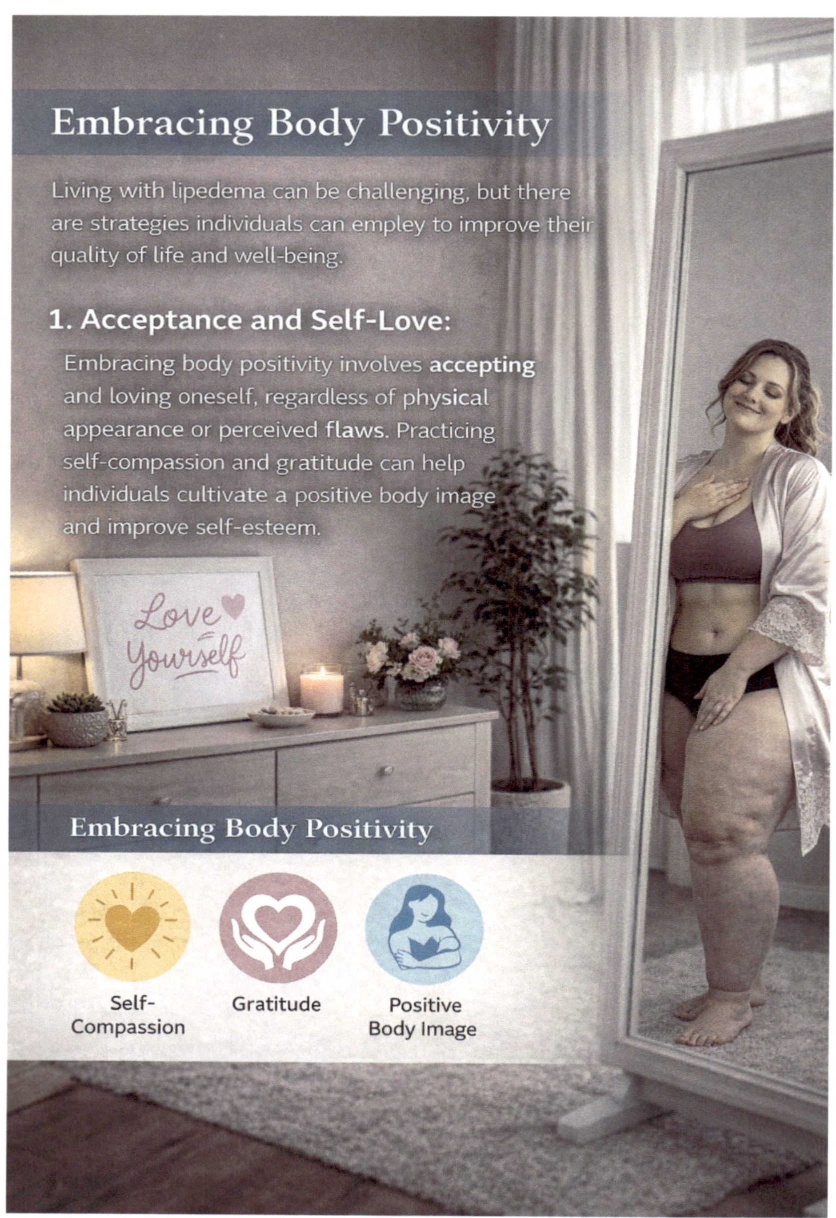

First and foremost, understanding lipedema is crucial. By recognizing the signs and symptoms, individuals can seek timely medical evaluation and diagnosis, ensuring appropriate management strategies are implemented early on. We've discussed the importance of embracing body positivity, practicing self-care, and building a supportive community. Connecting with others who understand the challenges of living with lipedema can provide invaluable emotional support and validation.

Treatment options for lipedema are varied, ranging from conservative measures such as lifestyle modifications and compression therapy to medical interventions like liposuction and lymphatic surgery. Each individual may require a tailored approach to treatment, guided by their unique symptoms, preferences, and healthcare provider recommendations.

Looking to the future, ongoing research holds promise for advancements in understanding the underlying mechanisms of lipedema, developing novel treatment modalities, and improving patient outcomes. By participating in research, advocating for increased awareness, and supporting initiatives aimed at advancing the field, individuals with lipedema can contribute to a brighter future for themselves and future generations.

In closing, living with lipedema is a journey filled with challenges, but it is also a journey of resilience, strength, and community. By staying informed, seeking support, and advocating for themselves, individuals with lipedema can lead fulfilling lives and inspire others along the way. Remember, you are not alone in your journey, and together, we can strive for a better understanding and management of lipedema.

Stay strong, stay empowered, and keep moving forward.

Warm regards.

9. Exploring Research Frontiers in Lipedema

Since we know that lipedema is a condition characterized by abnormal accumulation of fat, often misunderstood and underdiagnosed, has sparked a surge of curiosity among researchers and patients alike. This chapter delves into the diverse array of research questions, hypotheses, and innovative ideas emerging from the Lipedema community, as showcased by the Lipedema Foundation.

1. Journal Club Discussions:

One proactive approach to foster collaboration and knowledge sharing within the Lipedema research community is through journal club discussions. These forums serve as catalysts for networking, exchange of ideas, and acceleration of research endeavors. By dissecting the latest findings in an open-forum format, researchers aim to engage young investigators, thus expanding the research workforce and enhancing professional awareness.

2. Millimeter Wave Technology Investigation:

The potential application of millimeter wave technology, primarily used in TSA scanners, for screening Lipedema represents a novel avenue for exploration. While anecdotal reports suggest its efficacy in identifying Lipedema-affected regions, formal studies are lacking. Collaborative efforts with TSA could pave the way for innovative screening methodologies.

3. Lipedema and Idiopathic Intracranial Hypertension (IIH) Correlation:

Observations hint at a potential correlation between Lipedema and IIH, both predominantly affecting women and exhibiting estrogen-related characteristics. Research endeavors to unravel this connection could lead to improved diagnosis and treatment strategies for affected individuals.

4. Skin Changes in Lipedema Patients:

Reports of altered skin tanning and sunburning patterns among Lipedema patients pose intriguing questions about underlying biological factors. Investigating this phenomenon could shed light on dermatological aspects of Lipedema and its pathogenesis.

5. Lymph Fluid Stagnancy and Cholesterol Levels:

The relationship between lymphatic fluid stagnancy in Lipedema and cholesterol levels warrants exploration. Understanding this link could aid patients in communicating symptoms to healthcare providers and guide potential interventions.

6. Autoimmune and Genetic Hypothesis:

The autoimmune and genetic hypothesis proposes that surface molecules on Lipedema fat cells may trigger an immune response. Investigating these molecules and potential therapeutic antibodies could offer promising avenues for treatment.

7. Steroid Hormones and Lipedema Onset:

Anecdotal evidence suggests a possible link between steroid use and Lipedema onset in males. Comprehensive studies exploring the impact of long-term steroid use on tissue composition and lymphatic function are crucial for understanding this association.

8. Repurposed Drugs in Lipedema Treatment:

Investigations into repurposed drugs, such as GLP-1RA drugs and guaifenesin, offer insights into potential therapeutic interventions and underlying biological mechanisms in Lipedema.

9. Connective Tissue Disease and Environmental Exposures:

Exploring the role of environmental factors, including food additives and farm chemicals, in exacerbating connective tissue diseases like Lipedema underscores the importance of public health initiatives and regulatory measures.

10. Autophagy and Lipophagy in Lipedema:

Research into autophagy and lipophagy mechanisms holds promise for understanding adipose tissue metabolism in Lipedema. Large-scale studies involving patient participation are essential for elucidating these processes and evaluating their therapeutic potential.

11. Histotripsy for Nodule Disruption:

The application of histotripsy, a focused ultrasound technique, for disrupting fibrotic nodules in Lipedema presents a non-invasive therapeutic avenue. Collaborative efforts with medical institutions could pave the way for clinical trials and improved treatment modalities.

In summary, the diverse range of research inquiries highlighted in this chapter underscores the multifaceted nature of Lipedema and the pressing need for collaborative, multidisciplinary research endeavors to unravel its complexities and advance therapeutic interventions.

Additional Research Questions from

https://www.lipedema.org/ideadatabase

Research Question: Lipedema fat cells have surface molecules(or antigens) that characterize it from normal fat. A normal female(non lipedematous) has antibodies against these antigens which does not let these cells grow. But a woman with lipedema does not have these molecules in her body which allows for the exponential growth of this type of fat. Why a woman with lipedema does not have these antibodies might be attributed to genetics. These molecules might be upregulated by the hormonal changes that occur during puberty, pregnancy and menopause.
So according to this hypothesis, lipedema is an autoimmune and genetic condition.

Asked by: Person with Lipedema,"Healthcare Worker, Other"
Type: Patient Observation

Impact: If this research idea is true , isolating those antibodies and introducing them into a body with lipedema could potentially be a treatment (or even better,a cure). This could lead to an improved quality of life for those suffering from this disease

Supportive Research: https://link.springer.com/chapter/10.1007/0-306-46887-5_9

https://www.sciencedirect.com/science/article/abs/pii/S0006291X9899622X

Data Collection Method: Blood Samples,Lipoaspirate,Biopsy ,DNA

Research Question: I have had three male patients that I strongly suspect have

Lipedema. Two of which have mothers with Lipedema. The third was on prescribed steroids for three years to treat a different condition, and then had rapid weight gain afterwards that he has had great difficulty losing.

He does not have anyone in his family with Lipedema that he is aware of. He was thin prior to the steroids. He presents with tissue very similar to Lipedema that is concentrated in the thighs and around the knees, with nodules that become more apparent with weight loss. I want to know if male use of steroids can be an initiating factor for Lipedema, since it is known that steroids have an impact on men's hormones.

Asked by: Person with Lipedema,Occupational Therapist,Other

Impact: Men are less likely to be diagnosed with Lipedema, and are therefore at an even greater risk of going unnoticed in this particular field. Answering this question would potentially help anyone who may have to take prescribed hormones and help providers acknowledge additional risks associated with their use.

Investigation Method: Study of men and women before, during, and after long term prescription steroid use and the difference between normal weight/tissue gain associated with steroid use vs Lipedema tissue. Use of compression during steroid use and after to reduce risk of lymphatic congestion/swelling.

Data Collection Method: Questionnaires/Surveys,Interviews,Biopsy ,Live Human,Medical Records

Research Question: Steroid hormones regulate alternate splicing, which in turn has implications for adipogenesis.

Nature of Observation: Research Findings (Published),Research Findings

(Unpublished)

Impact: Understanding why adipocyte hypertorphy and hyperplaisia are occuring has implications for making the patients quality of life better, and may impact treatments.

Supportive Research: https://www.thieme-connect.com/products/ejournals/abstract/10.1055/s-2002-33249

References

1. Lipedema Foundation: The Lipedema Foundation is a non-profit organization dedicated to raising awareness, supporting research, and providing resources for individuals living with lipedema. Visit their website for information on treatment options, research updates, and support groups: [Lipedema Foundation](https://lipedema.org/)

2. National Organization for Rare Disorders (NORD): NORD offers comprehensive information on rare diseases, including lipedema. Their website provides an overview of lipedema, treatment options, and links to support groups: [NORD - Lipedema](https://rarediseases.org/rare-diseases/lipedema/)

3. PubMed: PubMed is a valuable resource for accessing medical literature and research articles on lipedema. Stay up-to-date with the latest advancements in lipedema research by searching for relevant articles and studies: [PubMed - Lipedema](https://pubmed.ncbi.nlm.nih.gov/?term=lipedema)

4. Lipedema Project: The Lipedema Project aims to educate patients and healthcare providers about lipedema through documentary films, educational materials, and advocacy efforts. Explore their website for educational resources and information on upcoming events: [Lipedema Project](https://www.lipedemaproject.org/)

5. International Lymphedema & Lipedema Society (ILF): The ILF provides education, resources, and support for individuals living with lymphedema and lipedema. Visit their website for information on treatment options, patient stories, and educational materials: [ILF](https://www.lipedema.org/)

These sources offer a wealth of information and support for individuals living with lipedema, as well as healthcare professionals and caregivers seeking to learn more about this condition.